HEALTHY LIFE TIPS AND AROMA THERAPY

ENGLISH EDITION

KAPILA SAINI

ISBN 978-1-68487-831-4

Contents

CHAPTER ONE

Introduction

*"Aware People about Health
Come on Let's make to World Healthy"*

Good health is a goal in itself. Only a healthy person can lead a happy and a good life. A healthy person is the basis of family, social welfare. But in the present environment, health is abundant in material resources.

Health is a very important subject. It is usually understood that being disease free is the definition of health. While being disease free is only one aspect of health and does not complete the definition of health.

The literal meaning of health is "to be in such a state of physical body in which you can perform all functions smoothly."

According to Gautam Buddha: Being healthy is the greatest gift for us. Health is the greatest wealth and the best relationship.

According to Gene Tunney: to enjoy the radiance of good health you must exercise.

According to Albert Einstein: Without health there is no life, but it is a state of sorrows and lethargy.

According to Anne Wilson Schaef: We can't buy good health, but it can be a very valuable savings account.

The question is what is health? When can we call a person healthy? It is generally believed that not having any type of physical and mental illness is health. But, apart from this in a healthy person, social, ideological, behavioral and ways of living all complete the definition of Health.

Human body is one of the best bodies among all creatures on this planet. It is better than any other species on the planet. But, maintaining the human body is also not easy. We must remember some things to be healty, otherwise we may also have to pay the price of life.

Any problem is not generated in a day or two. Not having a routine, not taking care of your diet, and similar things gradually cause these problems,

If we want to live a long and healthy life we will have to take care about small things in our daily routine.

For this you just need to give a small amount of time daily towards your health.

Just by remembring some important but simple things we can get a really big treasure of Health, so let's start and learn some health tips.

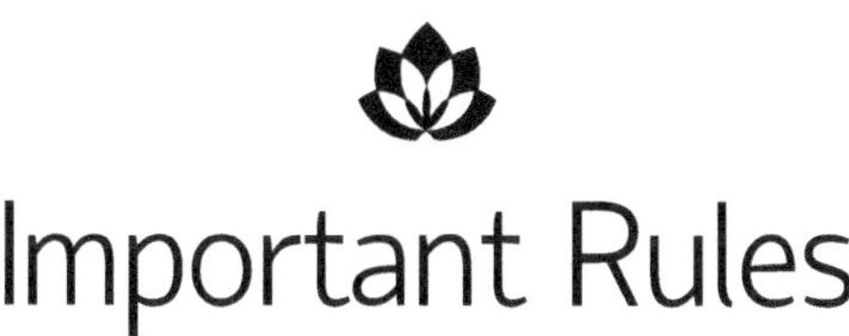

CHAPTER TWO

Important Rules

Exercise

Exercise is as important as food and water. By Exercising we stay healthy Physically and Mentally.

Benefits of Exercising

1. Muscles remain healthy: Along with healthy muscles, regular exercise also helps in smooth flow of blood. It also helps a lot to activate brain cells.
2. Calories are burnt: If you are gaining weight due to any reason and you want to control it, then your metabolism should be good for this. Exercising regularly improves metabolism and also burns calories, which keeps weight under control.
3. Relief from stress: Regular exercise also keeps the mind sharp. Regular exercise acts like a medicine for depression.
4. Blood pressure: Regular exercise reduces the problem of blood pressure. People who exercise daily, the problem of high BP is reduced by 75%. Aerobics G regulates blood pressure.
5. Cholesterol: Regular exercise reduces the amount of bad cholesterol in the body and increases the amount of good cholesterol. Exercise also keeps our heart healthy and oxygen level is also controlled.
6. Relief from pain: Those who have problems with pain in the back and extremities, they are benefited from regular exercise. If there is a feeling of weakness in the body, then exercise generates energy in the body. Regular exercise also increases immunity.

Balanced Diet

To stay healthy, we need a balanced diet because most of the diseases arise from wrong eating habits. Food is not made for the taste of our tongue, but food is made to meet our energy needs.

CHAPTER THREE

Eating Habits for Staying Healthy

1. Fruits or Salads: Eat a bowl of fruits or salads before meals, after which the food is easily digested and the nutrients present in them improve your health. They also help in fighting diseases. Immunity is also staffed by this. Fruits should always be kept at room temperature.

2. Make sure to have breakfast: Staying for a long time on an empty stomach in the morning is injurious to health. Apart from obesity, it also causes stomach diseases. By having breakfast regularly in the morning, you become healthy and energetic. In such a situation, even if you are not able to have lunch for any reason, then also energy remains in the body.

3. Drinking juice: Make a habit of drinking juice. By drinking orange juice with food, the body is able to absorb nutrients better. In addition, you can drink any juice you like. Sugar should not be added to it.

4. Fasting: Take a good diet every day but do fasting for 1 day in a week or 1 day in a month. By not eating food for 1 day, the metabolic rate increases, apart from this the risk of heart diseases is reduced by 40%.

5. Fruits: By making a habit of eating one fruit daily, you will start feeling energetic.

6. Brown instead of white: If you use brown bread instead of white in the food, brown rice instead of white rice, use wheat flour instead of maida, then it is beneficial for our health.

7. Salt intake: The amount of salt in the food should be balanced. We should avoid eating extra salt in food. Salt should not be put on top other than the amount of salt that has been added while cooking.

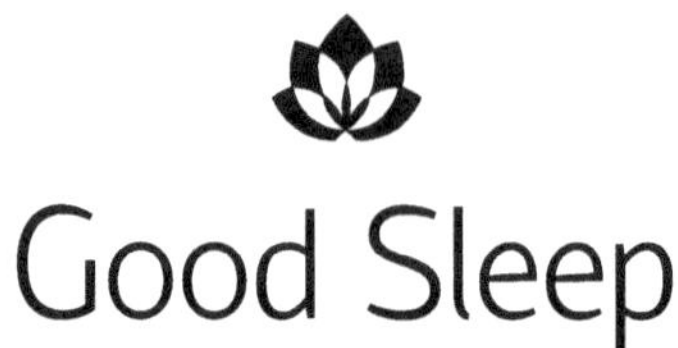

CHAPTER FOUR

Good Sleep

Just as a mother takes care of her child, in the same way the universe nourishes everyone by resting in the state of sleep. Sleep is a necessary and a natural part of our daily routine, sleep is essential for leading a healthy life. Deep and good and complete sleep gives complete rest to our body. Due to which the body gets freshness and energy. Weakness, irritability, tension, lethargy and short life problems arise due to incomplete sleep. That's why we need sleep at the right time and in plenty.

Some tips to get Good Sleep

1. First of all take deep breaths and meditate before sleeping.
2. Wash your feet before sleeping and massage with oil, it helps in good sleep.
3. Wear comfortable cotton clothes while sleeping, this allows air circulation in the body.
4. If you have trouble falling asleep, then you can drink mint juice mixed with water shortly before bedtime. If you are not able to sleep due to any stress or problem, then you can use Ashwagandha. You can also include cottage cheese in your diet, a chemical found in cottage cheese called tryptophan, which produces the neurotransmitter serotonin, helps in getting rid of the problem like lack of sleep from the body.

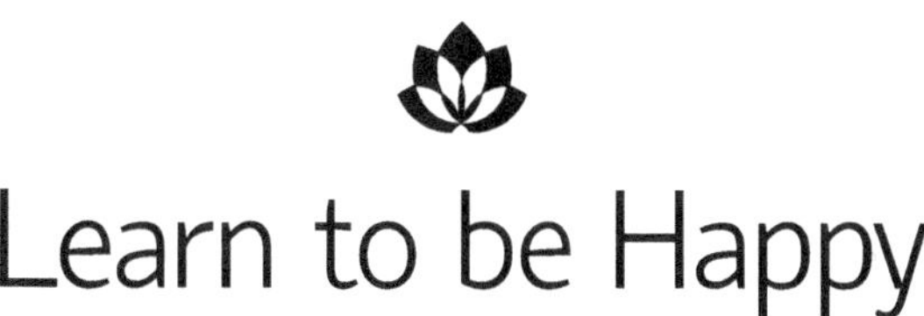

Learn to be Happy

There are many sorrows and pains in life, the question arises that how do you handle them. Know very well that your greatest wealth is your health and happiness of you and your family. If you want to be happy in life, then understand the bad habits of your body and mind, and try to remove them through yoga. Always think positive and learn to separate yourself from pain and sorrow. Your small effort will bring change in your life.

CHAPTER SIX

Always take care of Cleanliness

Cleanliness is closely related to everyone's life. Cleanliness keeps our health good. If our health will be good only then we will be able to adopt positive thinking in our life. That's why one should always take care of cleanliness. We should also take care of the internal cleanliness of the body.

We all know that infections spread due to dirt, so we should keep every part of the body clean.

1. Cleaning of nails: Cleanliness of nails is very important for us. Because we do all our work with our hands and if the nails are big and dirty then we are at increased risk of getting diseases. Since big nails are prone to dirt, always cut your nails on time and keep them clean.
2. Cleaning of hands: Along with cleaning the nails, care should be taken for the cleanliness of the hands. Because the dirt spreads through the hands in the food and then in the body by eating, so hands must be washed before preparing and eating food.
3. Cleaning the mouth: After waking up in the morning and before going to sleep at night, it is necessary to clean the teeth. By doing this you will stay away from any dental problems.
4. Cleansing of the skin: It is natural to have an infection due to sweating, so take a bath twice in the summers. Keep in mind, it is very important to get sweat out of our body. But it is equally important to clean the sweat. If we do not let sweat come out of our body, then that too is injurious to health.
5. Hair Cleaning: Hair cleaning should also not be ignored, because they make the beauty of the body. If you do not take care of the hair, then problems like dandruff, itching will arise from the head. That's why we

must apply oil once a week, so that the hair gets nourished and wash the hair twice a week.

6. Foot Cleaning: It is often seen that people make their whole body shine, but do not pay any attention to their feet. Due to which the heels start cracking and later they give pain and discomfort. Feet should be nicely cleaned every other day.

Excessive cleaning is also harmful

It's a good thing to keep your surroundings clean. In this way, many harmful bacteria and diseases stay away from us. But some people have such a craze for cleanliness that they do things like washing hands frequently, taking bath several times a day, mopping the house many times, repeatedly seeing dust particles everywhere, etc.

Actually it is a kind of thinking. According to psychologists, any person in whose mind the thought of cleaning takes home. So he keeps repeating it over and over again. This is called Obsessive Compulsive Disorder (OCD). Such people do not even know that the good bacteria that are needed also die by excessive cleaning. Then diseases arise because of that.

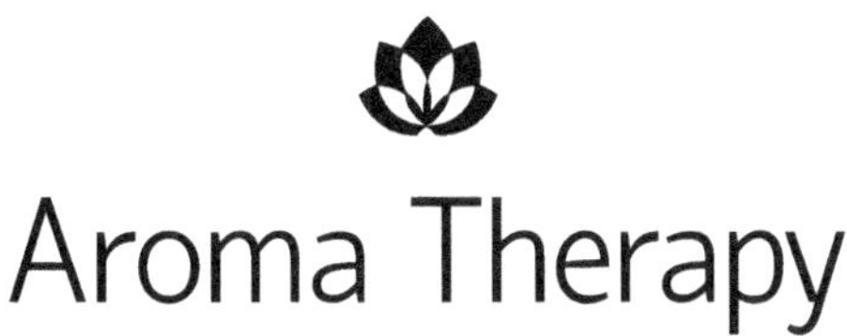

CHAPTER EIGHT

Aroma Therapy

According to Ayurveda, there are many such plants and vegetations around us which are very beneficial. The use of natural medicines has been going on since the days of our grandmothers.

Aroma means fragrance and therapy means healing. That is, aromatherapy is a formal medicinal process. In which important elements are extracted from many plants and it is used in the treatment of diseases. In this therapy, a variety of oils, water steam, some aromatic mixtures, etc., are used for massage and bathing. During therapy, the acupressure points on the body are massaged externally, which helps the body to relax.

What is Aroma Therapy?

In Aroma Therapy, diseases are treated through aroma. Aroma therapy is a very effective treatment for relieving stress and fatigue. Aromatherapy enhances brain function and strengthens the immune system. It does not cause any kind of allergy to the body. That is, it protects the body from diseases without harming it. In this, our brain, nervous system etc. are benefited by the fragrance. In this, fragrant things are included such as trees - plants, leaves, fruits - flowers, some vegetables and some spices, etc. In this, the extract of fruits and flowers is extracted by distillation method, it is called essential oil. And each extract has its own distinct aroma and identity. The treatment given with these extracts is called aromatherapy. The main oils used in aromatherapy are eucalyptus, geranium, lavender, rose, vermillion, jasmine, sandal, etc. Apart from oil, it is also available in the form of lotion, powder, clay mask, banding salt, facial streamer, cream, etc.

Health Benefits of Aroma Therapy

1. Prevention of stress: The natural fragrance of flowers makes us all happy. This is a great remedy to get rid of stress. If you often suffer from stress, aromatherapy can be a very beneficial treatment for you. With this treatment, your mind will be relaxed and peaceful and the stress will go away soon.

2. Energy transmission: Aroma therapy helps in circulation of energy throughout the body and activates the body. According to a report from the University of Petersburg, aromatherapy brings about changes in the human brain, fragrance not only changes the state of mind, but also relaxes and energizes the body. There are neurons in the brain that recognize scent, these neurons make the brain active due to aroma.

3. Natural Rejuvenation of the Skin: If your skin has become dry, your natural facial oil has been reduced. So aromatherapy is proven to be very effective. The oils used in it increase the antibacterial ability in our body. Due to which the problems related to the skin end quickly. The natural oils used in aromatherapy act as anti-bacterial agents in the body. This reduces scars and wrinkles caused by the injury. After aromatherapy, there is a special kind of softness in the skin.

Aroma therapy is used to maintain the health of both mind and body. This also solves many other problems.

1. Headache, migraine or body pain
2. Insomnia or other sleep problems
3. Stress, anxiety or mental stress
4. Joint Pain
5. Reducing the Side Effects of Chemotherapy
6. Minimizing discomfort during delivery
7. Boosts Immunity and Digestion

Products used for Aroma Therapy

1. Tea Tree Extract: This is very helpful in removing the problem of oily skin and acne. Along with increasing the volume of cells, it also cleans them. It works like magic on blemishes, acne and dark circles. Take a drop of tea tree oil with daily lotion or apply directly to the stained area.

2. Lavender: Rich in many medicinal properties. It is used in many ways. such as minor burns and sunburns, rashes, wounds and insect bites. It is also used to treat muscle and headache etc.

3. Peppermint: If you are feeling excessively hot during the summer days, then put a drop of peppermint oil in the water and massage it on the soles of the feet. So immediately the body temperature comes under control. It keeps the mind calm, apart from this, peppermint essential oil is very useful in headache, digestive system related problems, nasal congestion, etc.

4. Eucalyptus: Eucalyptus is a medicine used for the elderly. In older people, it will be beneficial to use it in case of fever, cold, muscle pain and stress in summer.

5. German Chemomile: This oil is very useful in summers. It is used for problems like burning, itching, tummy titis, lumps, acne, nappy rash, eczema and dry skin.

6. Sandalwood paste: To bring coolness in the mind, it is advised to apply sandalwood on the forehead. There is a mention of 11 senses in Ayurveda, in this the 11th sense is the mind and we make our mind healthy with fragrance. Healthy mind means positive thoughts, which is very necessary in today's environment.

7. Rose: The fragrance of rose gives peace in Pitra Dosha. Apart from stress, its aroma provides relief in digestion related problems. Pregnant women should not take the fragrance of roses.

www.ingramcontent.com/pod-product-compliance
Lightning Source LLC
Chambersburg PA
CBHW050713250726
48662CB00002B/1002